One month without sugar

Embrace the **SUGAR-ZERO** method and transform your body !

Table of contents

Chapter 1 : Understanding the
ravages of sugar on your body
5

Chapter 2 : The fundamentals of a
sugar-free diet
13

Chapter 3 : The 30-day sugar-free
challenge
23

Chapter 4 : SUGAR-ZERO
43

Chapter 5 : Sugar and athletic
performance
51

Chapter 6 : Sugar and women's health
58

Chapter 7 : Sugar and parenting
66

Chapter 8 : Sugar and blood sugar
75

Chapter 9 : Sugar and longevity
83

Chapter 10 : Living a sugar-free life after the challenge
90

PROGRESS JOURNAL
99

Chapter 1 : Understanding the ravages of sugar on your body

Discover the detrimental effects of sugar on your health and how it can harm your overall well-being.

Sugar, that delicious little indulgence we add to our food and drinks, may seem harmless, even essential for flavoring our lives. However, behind its deceptive sweetness, sugar hides consequences far more detrimental to our health than we could imagine. In this first chapter, we will explore the havoc that sugar can wreak on our bodies, on our quest for a healthy and balanced life. First and foremost, it's important to understand that sugar is a real explosive for our energy levels.

When we consume foods high in sugar, our body goes into a frenzy of insulin production to lower our blood sugar level. This insulin spike then leads to a dramatic drop in our energy, often leaving us tired and lethargic. A life without sugar allows us to maintain a more stable energy throughout the day, thus avoiding the highs and lows of a sugary diet.

Beyond its impact on our energy level, sugar can also be a catalyst for more serious health problems. Studies have shown that excessive sugar consumption is linked to obesity, type 2 diabetes, and other chronic diseases such as cardiovascular diseases. By limiting our sugar intake, we therefore take control of our health and significantly reduce the risks of developing these conditions.

But how can sugar harm our general well-being ?
Firstly, it can *disrupt our hormonal balance.* When we consume foods high in sugar, our body releases dopamine, a neurotransmitter often associated with the feeling of pleasure. Unfortunately, this dopamine rush can create an addiction, pushing us to seek more sugar to achieve the same effect. Ultimately, this can weaken our willpower and affect our ability to make healthy decisions.

Moreover, sugar can also alter our mood. Some studies have suggested that excessive sugar intake can exacerbate symptoms of anxiety and depression. This is partly due to how sugar affects our blood sugar levels. When we consume high-sugar foods, our blood sugar spikes quickly, then drops rapidly afterward. These fluctuations can impact our emotional state, sometimes leaving us feeling anxious and depressed.

By becoming aware of the detrimental effects of sugar on our body and our overall well-being, we take the first step towards a healthier and more balanced life. It is crucial to understand that we have the power to change our eating habits and to adopt a more mindful approach to our sugar consumption.

We will explore the different steps to adopt the **SUGAR-ZERO** method, a practical and effective approach to reduce our sugar intake and positively transform our lives.

Now that we are aware of the detrimental effects of sugar on our body and overall well-being, it's time to take action. How can we adopt a sugar-free approach and reap all its benefits ?

Here are the key steps to help you start your journey towards a sugar-free life.

First, **it's important to review our eating habits**. Take the time to identify foods that are high in sugar and are an integral part of your daily diet. Sodas, sweet desserts, confectioneries, and processed products are typically the biggest sources of sugar. Make an effort to reduce or completely avoid these foods, and replace them with healthier, natural alternatives.

Next, **learn to read nutritional labels**. Sugar can hide under different names such as corn syrup, maltodextrin, dextrose, or inverted sugar. Familiarize yourself with these terms and be vigilant about their presence in the products you buy. Opt for unprocessed foods and favor foods high in fiber, protein, and healthy fats.

Another important step is to **moderate your consumption of simple carbohydrates**. Even foods considered healthy can be high in sugar. Fruits, for example, naturally contain sugar, but they are also an important source of vitamins and fibers. Learn to choose fruits with low sugar content like berries and citrus, and limit your intake of sweeter fruits like bananas and grapes.

As part of the **SUGAR-ZERO** method, it's also crucial to reduce your consumption of added sugar. Sweeten your food and drinks with natural alternatives such as stevia, xylitol, or pure maple syrup. These alternatives allow you to satisfy your sweet tooth while avoiding the harmful effects of sugar on your health.

Finally, don't forget to stay motivated and surround yourself with support. Adopting a sugar-free life can be a challenge, but remember the benefits for your overall well-being. Set realistic goals and celebrate each small victory. Inform your family and friends of your approach and seek their encouragement. You can also look for online communities or local support groups to share your experiences and get additional advice.

Chapter 2 : The fundamentals of a sugar-free diet

Learn the basics of a sugar-free diet and the foods to favor to promote a healthier life.

The SUGAR-ZERO method, which we'll discuss throughout this book, is an innovative approach aimed at significantly reducing our sugar intake. You'll be surprised to see how much this can transform your life, whether in terms of your energy, weight, mood, and overall well-being.

Before diving into practical advice, it's important to understand what a sugar-free diet really entails. Contrary to what some might think, it's not just about cutting out candies, pastries, and sodas from your diet. A sugar-free diet goes well beyond that.

Firstly, it's crucial to differentiate between added sugars and sugars naturally present in foods. Added sugars are often found in processed foods such as sweetened beverages, sauces, cereals, and even so-called "healthy" products. These sugars are quickly digested by our body, causing a rapid increase in our blood sugar level, followed by a sharp drop that leaves us tired and hungry.

On the other hand, sugars naturally present in fruits, vegetables, and dairy products are not harmful to our health when consumed in the right proportions. These foods also contain fibers, vitamins, minerals, and antioxidants essential for our well-being.

In the first half of this chapter, we'll focus on the foods to favor to adopt a healthy sugar-free diet. Here are some suggestions to get you started :

1. **Vegetables** are your best friends : opt for a wide variety of fresh and colorful vegetables. They are rich in nutrients, fibers, and antioxidants, without adding unwanted sugar to your diet.

2. **Fruits in moderation** : although fruits are naturally sweet, they can be consumed in reasonable amounts as part of a balanced diet. Choose fresh, seasonal fruits, and favor low glycemic index options like berries, apples, and pears.

3. **Lean proteins** : proteins are essential for our health and satiety. Opt for lean sources such as chicken, turkey, fish, eggs, and legumes.

4. **Healthy fats** : don't shy away from healthy fats found in avocados, nuts, seeds, and vegetable oils like olive oil. They are important for our heart health and brain.

5. **Whole grains** : when choosing carbohydrates, opt for whole grains such as quinoa, brown rice, and oats. They are rich in fibers and nutrients.

6. **Low-sugar dairy products** : if you consume dairy products, prefer options without added sugar or low in sugar. Choose plant-based milk or natural yogurts that you can sweeten yourself with fruits.

By following these basic recommendations, you will begin to gradually eliminate sugar from your diet while nourishing yourself in a balanced and nourishing way.

Remember that every small step counts, and the benefits you'll reap from adopting a sugar-free diet will delight both your body and mind.

Here are some additional fundamental tips to start your sugar-free month :

- **Minimize processed foods** : One of the first steps to adopting a sugar-free diet is to avoid processed foods as much as possible. These products are often high in added sugars, saturated fats, and harmful additives for our health. Read package labels carefully and avoid foods that contain hidden sugars under names like corn syrup, fructose, dextrose, or sucrose. Always prefer raw and natural foods without hesitation.

- **Get creative in the kitchen** : Adopting a sugar-free diet doesn't mean you have to deprive yourself of flavors and gustatory pleasures. On the contrary, it invites you to be creative in the kitchen ! Experiment with new recipes using natural sugar alternatives such as stevia, pure maple syrup, raw honey, and dried fruits. You'll be surprised at how delightful sugar-free eating can be.

- **Opt for healthy snacks** : Snacks are often a major source of sugar in our diet. Instead of snacking on chocolate bars or sugary cookies, choose healthier alternatives like almonds, nuts, seeds, or vegetables cut into sticks with a dip made from natural yogurt and fresh herbs. These snacks will provide you with essential nutrients and help maintain your energy throughout the day.

- **Eat at regular times** : Eating at regular times can play a significant role in managing your sugar intake. Establish a regular schedule for meals and snacks to avoid cravings that might lead you to consume sugary foods. Planning your meals in advance also gives you a better idea of healthy foods you can incorporate into your diet.

- **Learn to decode product labels** : When shopping, take the time to carefully read product labels.

Manufacturers can be cunning by using misleading terms to hide the presence of sugar. Familiarize yourself with the different names of sugar and the many ingredients that may contain it. This will enable you to make more informed choices and find healthier alternatives.

- **Find support** : Adopting a sugar-free diet can sometimes be challenging, especially when those around us continue to consume sugary foods. Don't hesitate to seek support from online support groups, forums, or even friends who share the same goal as you. Sharing your experiences, tips, and recipes can be a source of motivation and inspiration to maintain your commitment to a sugar-free life.

Remember, every small step counts ! Even the decision to eliminate one spoonful of sugar from your coffee each morning is a step in the right direction. Continue to persevere and stay motivated to transform your life day by day.

Chapter 3 : The 30-day sugar-free challenge

"*You are what you eat.*" This famous quote by Hippocrates perfectly summarizes the importance of our diet in our quality of life. Sugar, in particular, has a major impact on our health and well-being.

So, it's time to embark on the 30-day sugar-free challenge ! Get ready to transform your life !

Week 1 : Stop & Uncover

At the beginning of this journey towards a sugar-free life, it's imperative to make a clean break with our previous habits. This first week is crucial; it lays the foundation for lasting transformation.

We'll start by identifying and eliminating the obvious sources of sugar in our daily lives, then venture to uncover those hidden where we least expect them.

Day 1 to 3 : Let's cut out direct sugar

During these first days, the goal is to stop all direct sugar consumption cold turkey. This means not adding sugar to your morning coffee or tea, nor giving in to the temptation of those sweet treats that catch our eye. The challenge is significant, but it's crucial for reeducating our palate and beginning to reduce our sugar dependence.

It's also time to become a nutritional detective.
Read the labels on everything you consume. You'll be surprised to find the amount of added sugar in products where you wouldn't expect it: from sandwich bread to tomato sauces, to breakfast cereals. This awareness is the first step towards deep change.

Day 4 to 7 : Discovering hidden sources

Now that direct sugar addition is behind us, it's time to tackle the hidden sources.

This approach requires adopting a more analytical perspective of our diet.

Start by keeping a food diary, noting everything you eat. This practice might seem tedious at first but will quickly prove to be a valuable tool for identifying unsuspected sugar sources.

Examine your eating habits closely: prepared meals, ready-made sauces, dressings, or even some so-called "health" products can contain significant amounts of added sugar.

The goal of this approach is twofold.

On one hand, it allows you to become aware of the sugary traps hidden in your diet. On the other hand, it prepares you to make more informed choices in the weeks to come.

These first days represent a real turning point. By giving up added sugar, you begin to rediscover the real taste of food, appreciate the natural flavor of fruits, vegetables, and even the more subtle taste of whole grains. This adjustment of your palate is essential for fully appreciating the changes to come.

Week 2 : Choose & Replace

As we progress on our journey towards a life free of sugar, the second week marks a crucial step: that of conscious and thoughtful substitution. Having already become aware of the sources of sugar, both obvious and hidden, we will now learn to choose healthy alternatives and replace sugar in our daily diet.

This phase is not just about restriction but also a wonderful opportunity for culinary rediscovery.

Day 8 to 14 : Choosing healthy alternatives

The challenge these days is to rethink our way of snacking and satisfying our sweet tooth. Instead of turning to sugary snacks, let's choose whole fruits. Fruits, with their fibers, vitamins, and minerals, not only nourish our bodies but also stabilize our blood sugar, thus reducing sweet cravings.

Incorporating whole grains into our meals also contributes to a more lasting feeling of fullness and a more constant energy supply throughout the day.

The goal here is twofold : not only are we reducing our sugar intake, but we are also improving our diet in general, making it richer in nutrients and beneficial components for our health.

Day 8 to 14 : Replacing sugar in our recipes

This week is also the perfect time to explore our culinary creativity. In cooking, sugar often plays a role more important than that of just a sweetener; it can affect the texture, color, and even preservation of food.

Fortunately, there are many natural alternatives that can fulfill these functions without the drawbacks of refined sugar.

Using spices like cinnamon, nutmeg, or vanilla can enrich our dishes with a depth of flavor without adding sugar. These spices can transform a bland dish into a complex and satisfying culinary creation. In recipes requiring a sweetener, fruit purees such as bananas, dates, or apples offer natural sweetness while providing additional fibers and nutrients.

Experimentation is the keyword this week. Each modified recipe, every successful substitution, is a small victory in our quest for a balanced and conscious diet. It's time to explore new flavors, play with textures, and discover that, yes, a rich and varied culinary world exists beyond sugar.

At the end of this second week, we not only start to see the first benefits of this transition on our health and energy, but we also open the door to a universe of flavors and culinary possibilities hitherto unexplored.

This journey of discovery will continue to enrich us well beyond these 30 days, transforming our relationship with food in a lasting and positive way.

Week 3 : Engage

Entering the third week of our SUGAR-ZERO journey, we approach a critical phase : commitment.

After reducing our sugar intake and exploring healthy alternatives, it's time to solidify these new habits and fully integrate them into our daily life. This week, the focus is on adopting new routines and social engagement, allowing us not only to support our changes but also to inspire those around us.

Day 15 to 21 : Engage in new routines

Regular physical activity plays an essential role in reducing sugar cravings.

Exercise not only helps burn calories; it also improves our mood and resilience to stress, thus reducing the temptations to turn to sugar for temporary comfort.

Incorporate a form of physical activity that you truly enjoy, whether it's a daily walk, yoga, swimming, or any other activity that gets you moving and brings you joy. Making exercise an integral part of your daily routine is a step further towards a balanced and sugar-free lifestyle.

Exploring cooking and experimenting with new no-added-sugar recipes is another way to reinforce your commitment.

Discovering delicious, nutritious, and added-sugar-free dishes and snacks can be incredibly rewarding.

Not only does it enrich your culinary repertoire, but it can also transform your relationship with food, making it more mindful and focused on your body's true needs.

Day 15 to 21 : Engage socially without sugar

It's also important to engage socially in our endeavor. Sharing our journey with friends or family, suggesting activities that don't revolve around food, or even initiating group sugar-free challenges can greatly strengthen our resolve and create a sense of community and support.

Sharing your discoveries, whether in the form of recipes, tips, or simply stories of your experiences, can inspire others to reflect on their sugar consumption and, potentially, to follow in your footsteps.

This group dynamic can not only provide you with additional support but also reinforce your own commitment by positioning you as a positive role model.

This week is dedicated to solidifying your new habits for the long term, through healthy routines and social engagement.

These actions strengthen your resilience against sugary temptations and promote a lasting transition towards a balanced lifestyle, free from sugar's grip.

By fully committing, both personally and socially, you pave the way for lasting well-being, emphasizing the importance of self-care while inspiring and supporting others in their journey.

Week 4 : Zero Excuses, Routines, Observations (ZERO)

The final stage of our journey leads us to consolidation and reflection. After three weeks of discovery, learning, and commitment, we arrive at a time to validate our efforts and introspect.

This week is dedicated to anchoring our new eating habits and becoming aware of the positive changes that have occurred, both physically and mentally.

Day 22 to 28 : Zero Excuses

Now is the time to face the final challenges with courage and determination. Temptations may arise, especially in social situations or moments of stress. However, armed with our new knowledge and habits, we are better equipped to face them without succumbing to sugar.

Use your food diary as a strategic tool to anticipate these situations and plan in advance. Identify moments when you are most vulnerable to sugar cravings and prepare strategies to effectively manage them.

Adopting a "zero excuses" approach does not mean being perfect at all times but rather having a firm will not to let small slip-ups become habits.

It's about recognizing the progress made and staying true to your commitment to a healthier lifestyle, remembering why you started this journey.

Day 29 to 30 : Routines and Observations

The last two days are for reflection and future planning. Take time to observe the changes in your body and mind.

Many report better energy, improved sleep, enhanced concentration, and general well-being.

Reflect on how these changes have influenced your daily life, your interactions with others, and your self-esteem.

Establish new eating routines that exclude added sugar as your new norm.

Consider how you can maintain these habits in the long term and continue to explore new ways to enjoy a healthy and balanced diet.
The end of these 30 days is not the end of the journey but rather the beginning of a new chapter in your life, where sugar no longer has the power to dictate your food choices.

You've gained the tools, knowledge, and most importantly, the confidence to continue on this path.

Keep applying the principles of the SUGAR-ZERO method, restart, inform yourself about the best foods to consume, discover new recipes, an activity to start alone or with friends, adapt, and learn.

The most important thing is to celebrate your successes, learn from your challenges, and always move towards a healthier and more fulfilled life.

Chapter 4 : SUGAR-ZERO

The SUGAR-ZERO journey we have embarked on together over these four weeks is much more than just an attempt to reduce sugar consumption.

It's a personal revolution, a profound redefinition of our relationship with food, accompanied by a tangible improvement in our physical and mental well-being.

This journey has allowed us to deconstruct our habits, uncover hidden sources of sugar, adopt healthy alternatives, engage in new routines, and ultimately redefine our diet around awareness and informed choice.

Key learnings and benefits

Increased food awareness : We've learned to read labels carefully and identify hidden sugars in our diet, enabling us to make more informed choices.

Culinary discovery : By replacing sugar with natural alternatives and incorporating whole grains and whole fruits into our diet, we've not only enriched our flavor palette but also increased our intake of essential nutrients.

Physical benefits : Reducing sugar consumption has led to better energy management throughout the day, improved sleep quality, and often, an improvement in body composition.

Mental and emotional resilience : Taking on this challenge has strengthened our willpower and discipline, equipping us with better management of sugar cravings and the emotions often linked to them.

Solidarity and social support : By sharing our journey, we've not only reinforced our own commitments but also inspired those around us to reflect on their sugar consumption.

Now, armed with this knowledge and these new habits, it is essential not to see the end of these 30 days as a conclusion but as the beginning of a sustainable lifestyle.

Here are some ways to continue on this path :

Continue exploring : The world of healthy eating is vast. Keep exploring new recipes, unfamiliar foods, and sugar alternatives. Learning is an endless journey.

Be kind to yourself : If you occasionally give in to a sugar craving, don't see it as a failure but as an opportunity to learn and better understand your triggers.

Involve those around you : Continue sharing your experience and encouraging a family and social environment that supports healthy eating. Organize meals where everyone brings a no-added-sugar dish, share your discoveries, and create new culinary traditions together.

Adopt a holistic view : Consider food not only as a source of pleasure and nutrition but also as a key component of your overall well-being. Integrate physical activity, mindfulness, and proper hydration as complementary pillars of your health.

Here is a table of snacks that usually tempt us during the day and their much healthier equivalents.

SWEET SNACKS	ALTERNATIVES
Soda	Sparkling water & lemon
Chocolate bar	Dark chocolate (70%) or handful of nuts
Ice Cream	Frozen fruits then blended
Donuts	Oat and banana muffins
Sweetened yogurt	Plain yogurt with honey
Packaged fruit juice	Whole fruit or homemade juice
Energy drinks	Tea, coffee

SWEET SNACKS	ALTERNATIVES
Flavored milk	Almond or coconut milk
Candies	Fruit slice, dried fruits
Sweetened dairy dessert	Cottage cheese, fruits & maple syrup
Breakfast cereals	Whole grain, sugar-free cereals
Sweetened fizzy drinks	Kombucha
Brioche	Whole grain bread with seeds

SWEET SNACKS	ALTERNATIVES
Sweetened fruit chips	Homemade dehydrated fruit chips
Syrups	Flavored water with herbs & fruit

Chapter 5 : Sugar and athletic performance

Explore how sugar can impact your athletic performance and discover strategies to optimize your energy without added sugar.

As a passionate athlete, you understand the importance of every aspect of your life that can influence your performance.

From regular training and proper nutrition to recovery and lifestyle, every detail counts towards achieving your sports goals. However, did you know that the amount of sugar you consume can also play a crucial role in your performance ?

Sugar has long been considered a quick energy source for athletes. After all, who hasn't grabbed a chocolate bar before an intense workout or competition ? These sweet snacks seemed to provide an instant energy boost, but at what cost ?

The truth is, excessive sugar consumption can actually be detrimental to your body and athletic performance. When you consume high-sugar foods, your body releases insulin to regulate your blood sugar level.

However, this can lead to a sudden and sharp drop in your energy, leaving you tired and lacking the reserves to continue performing at your best.

Moreover, excessive sugar consumption can also impact your weight, endurance, and recovery. Added sugars in many processed foods can lead to unwanted weight gain, making you less agile on the field. Additionally, sugar can cause inflammation in your body, slowing down your recovery process after intense training.

If you want to optimize your athletic performance and adopt a healthier lifestyle, it's time to reconsider your relationship with sugar.

Adopting the SUGAR ZERO method will allow you to find healthier alternatives and optimize your energy without added sugar.

Hydration plays a key role in your athletic performance. Avoid sugary drinks and opt for water or natural energy drinks like coconut water.

Hydrate regularly before, during, and after exercise to maintain your energy at its peak.

By reducing the amount of added sugar in your diet, you can significantly optimize your athletic performance.

Prepare to experience a noticeable increase in your endurance, recover faster, and have constant energy throughout your workouts.

Don't forget green vegetables in your meals, such as spinach and broccoli, which are rich in essential nutrients and fiber, helping to regulate your blood sugar level. Incorporate them into your meals or prepare green smoothies for a natural energy boost before training.

Another key strategy to optimize your performance without added sugar is to plan your meals and snacks in a balanced way. Ensure to include lean proteins, complex carbohydrates, and healthy fats in every meal to maintain a constant energy level. For example, before a workout, you might opt for grilled chicken with vegetables and quinoa rather than sugar-rich pasta.

After exercising, prefer protein-rich foods to aid muscle recovery, such as Greek yogurt or salmon.

Regarding training, a sugar-free approach doesn't mean you have to reduce the intensity or duration of your sessions. On the contrary, by adopting a balanced diet and avoiding added sugars, you can optimize your performance.

It's also important to consider your individual energy needs. Some people may need more carbohydrates to support their training, while others may benefit from a diet richer in healthy fats. Experiment and listen to your body to determine what works best for you.

Finally, don't forget to rest and recover adequately after your training sessions. Quality sleep, stress management, and relaxation are all important factors in maintaining a balance in your athletic life.

In conclusion, by adopting the 30-day SUGAR ZERO method, you can maximize your athletic performance without added sugar. By adjusting your diet to include protein-rich and fiber-rich foods, choosing natural hydrating drinks, and planning your meals in a balanced way, you will optimize your energy and endurance.

Each individual is unique, and it's important to experiment to find the approach that suits you best. Take care of your body and mind, and you'll be ready to face every sports challenge with confidence and vitality.

Chapter 6 : Sugar and women's health

It's no longer a secret that sugar, this sweet temptation that appears in various forms, is omnipresent in our daily lives.

However, did you know that its excessive consumption can have a significant impact on health, particularly women's health ?

The harmful effects of sugar on health are numerous and particularly concerning for women. Indeed, excessive sugar consumption can lead to hormonal imbalances, blood sugar disorders, weight gain, and even fertility issues.

Hormones are the engine of our body, playing a crucial role in women's health.

Unfortunately, sugar can disrupt this delicate balance. When we consume high-sugar foods, our blood sugar levels rise rapidly, causing insulin to be released into the body. This insulin overload can lead to hormonal fluctuations, resulting in imbalances such as polycystic ovary syndrome (PCOS), menstrual disorders, and even early menopause.

Moreover, excessive sugar consumption can lead to weight gain, especially in the abdominal region. This accumulation of visceral fat is not only linked to an increased risk of cardiovascular diseases but also to fertility issues in women.

It is therefore essential for women to be aware of the impact of sugar on their health and to adopt healthier eating habits. Here are some specific tips for women seeking a better quality of life :

- **Reduce your added sugar consumption** : Avoid sugary drinks and processed foods that often contain high amounts of hidden sugar. Favor natural foods and healthier sweet alternatives, such as fresh fruits.

- **Consume complex carbohydrates** : Choose foods rich in fiber, such as vegetables, whole grains, and legumes. These foods release sugar gradually into the blood, avoiding blood sugar spikes.

- **Favor healthy fats** : Healthy fats, such as those found in avocados, nuts, and seeds, are essential for hormonal balance and satiety. They will help you reduce your sugar cravings.

- **Engage in regular physical activity** : Regular exercise not only helps maintain a healthy weight but also helps regulate blood sugar and balance hormones. Find an activity you enjoy and integrate it into your routine.

In conclusion, sugar can have a considerable impact on women's health, leading to hormonal imbalances, blood sugar disorders, weight gain, and fertility issues. It is crucial for women to take steps to reduce their sugar consumption and adopt a healthier diet.

The harmful effects of sugar on women's health are not limited to what has been presented. In reality, excessive consumption can also impact women's cardiovascular health and increase their risk of developing lifestyle-related diseases.

Women are already faced with specific health risks regarding heart health, especially after menopause. Hormones play a significant role in regulating cholesterol, and when this balance is disturbed by sugar, it can lead to an increase in LDL cholesterol ("bad" cholesterol) and a decrease in HDL cholesterol ("good" cholesterol).

Furthermore, excessive sugar consumption can contribute to chronic inflammation, a major risk factor for cardiovascular diseases. When our body is constantly exposed to high levels of sugar, it can lead to oxidative stress, an imbalance of antioxidants, and an increase in the production of inflammatory molecules.

It is therefore essential for women to take steps to reduce their sugar consumption and adopt a healthier lifestyle to prevent cardiovascular diseases. Here are some additional tips to help you achieve this goal :

- **Increase your consumption of antioxidant-rich foods**: Antioxidants can help protect your body against damage caused by oxidative stress. Colorful fruits and vegetables, such as berries, leafy greens, and citrus, are particularly rich in antioxidants.

- **Limit your alcohol consumption** : Excessive alcohol consumption can not only increase your sugar intake but also be linked to an increased risk of cardiovascular diseases. Limit yourself to moderate consumption, or abstain entirely if you can.

- **Manage your stress** : Chronic stress can have a negative impact on cardiovascular health. Find stress management techniques that work for you, such as meditation, yoga, or therapy.

- **Regularly check your cholesterol levels** : It's important to monitor your cholesterol levels regularly to detect any increases that could be linked to excessive sugar consumption. If necessary, talk to your doctor about steps to maintain healthy cholesterol.

Chapter 7 : Sugar and parenting

Explore how sugar can impact your family's health and discover tips for adopting a sugar-free diet for children.

Parenting is an exciting and challenging adventure, and one of these challenges is undoubtedly our children's diet. As parents, we want to give them the best start in life, which includes a balanced and healthy diet. Unfortunately, in our modern society, sugar has insidiously infiltrated our lives and our children's.

This sweet temptation is everywhere, from breakfast cereals to biscuits and sodas. It's difficult to escape this sugary allure, especially when our children are exposed to enticing advertisements and social pressures. But it's time to take control and protect our family's health.

Excessive sugar consumption can have serious repercussions on our children's health. Besides the risk of obesity and dental caries, sugar can also affect their concentration and energy. Many parents complain about their children's hyperactivity, not realizing that sugar can be the main cause. By limiting their sugar intake, we can offer them a better quality of life.

So, how can we adopt a sugar-free diet for children? Here are some tips to help you on this wonderful journey :

- **Educate and raise awareness** : Start by explaining to your children the dangers of sugar to their health. Involve them in the decision-making process by showing them healthier alternatives and explaining why it's important to reduce their sugar consumption.

- **Cook together** : Involve your children in meal and snack preparation. Cooking together is an excellent way to teach them to appreciate natural foods and discover new flavors. Opt for sugar-free recipes, using natural sweeteners like honey or fruits.

- **Make smart choices** : When shopping, teach your children to read food labels. Avoid processed foods high in sugar and favor fresh, unprocessed foods. Choose fruits, vegetables, whole grains, and lean proteins.

- **Reinvent desserts** : Desserts are an integral part of our diet, but they don't have to be filled with sugar. Explore healthy and delicious alternatives, like fruit-based desserts or dark chocolate. Many sugar-free recipes are available online to satisfy the taste buds of the entire family.

- **Be a role model** : As always, children learn a lot by example. Show them that you too are willing to give up excessive sugar consumption. Adopt a balanced diet and encourage them to do the same.

By implementing these tips, you can help your family adopt a sugar-free diet, which will have long-term health benefits. You'll be surprised at how well your children can adapt and enjoy a healthier diet.

Facing resistance and difficulties

Although adopting a sugar-free diet for children can bring many health benefits, it doesn't mean the change will be easy. It's important to recognize and address the resistances and difficulties that may arise.

First, it's essential to understand that children may be reluctant to give up their favorite sugary foods. They may express discontent, feel deprived, and even actively resist these changes. This is where your communication and patience as a parent play a crucial role.

Try to explain to your children why you want to reduce their sugar intake in a clear and understandable way. By showing them images, videos, or stories about the harmful effects of sugar on health, you can further raise their awareness and help them understand your decision.

Then, involve them in the decision-making process. Ask for their opinions on the healthier alternatives you propose and encourage them to participate in preparing sugar-free meals and snacks. By giving them a sense of control and responsibility, they'll be more inclined to accept these changes.

It's also important to be creative when it comes to cooking sugar-free meals for your children. Explore new recipes and discover delicious fruit-based desserts or dark chocolate treats together. Make it a fun experience and discover new flavors with your children.

When shopping, resist the temptation of processed foods high in sugar. Teach your children to read food labels and make smart choices. Explain why it's better to choose fresh and unprocessed foods, such as fruits, vegetables, whole grains, and lean proteins.

Remember, you are a role model for your children. Show them that you're willing to give up excessive sugar consumption by adopting a balanced diet yourself. Encourage them to join you in this adventure and make healthy choices.

Lastly, be patient. The process of adapting to a sugar-free diet may take time. Your children may not immediately embrace the changes, but don't get discouraged. Continue offering them healthy alternatives and reminding them of the health benefits, and they will eventually get used to this new way of eating.

By adopting a sugar-free diet for children, you're making a decision that will significantly impact their long-term health. Following the tips presented in this chapter, you can help your family reduce its sugar intake and adopt a balanced and healthy diet.

Remember, every small action counts. By cooking together, making smart food choices, reinventing desserts, and being a role model for your children, you can make a positive difference in their lives.

Be prepared to face challenges and resistance, as each step towards a sugar-free diet is a step towards a healthier and more fulfilling life for your family.

Chapter 8 : Sugar and *blood sugar*

Understand how sugar influences your blood sugar levels and discover strategies for maintaining optimal sugar levels in your body.

Sugar is ubiquitous in our daily lives. From enticing pastries to sweetened drinks, and delicious desserts, our modern society is flooded with sugary temptations. However, it's crucial to understand how sugar can influence our blood sugar levels and, consequently, our overall health.

To start, it's important to know what blood sugar is. Simply put, it refers to the amount of sugar (*glucose*) present in our blood. When we consume foods high in sugar, our blood sugar levels increase, triggering the release of insulin from our pancreas. Insulin allows glucose to enter our cells and be used as an energy source.

However, excessive sugar consumption can lead to unhealthy fluctuations in our blood sugar levels. When we consume high-sugar foods, our body is overwhelmed with glucose, resulting in a larger release of insulin. These insulin spikes can cause a rapid drop in our blood sugar levels, leaving us tired, hungry, and unable to concentrate.

Besides these unwanted energy fluctuations, excessive sugar

consumption can also have long-term health consequences. Studies have shown that a diet high in sugar is linked to an increased risk of developing diseases such as type 2 diabetes, obesity, heart disease, and even some types of cancer.

Now that we understand how sugar influences our blood sugar, it's time to discover strategies for maintaining optimal sugar levels in our body.

Firstly, it's crucial to monitor our sugar intake. Carefully read food product labels and be aware of the amount of added sugar in processed foods. Opt instead for natural, unprocessed foods, rich in fiber, which allow for a slower absorption of sugar into the blood.

Additionally, learn to recognize the different names of sugar present in food products. Be mindful of these terms when choosing your foods.

Moreover, prefer foods with a low glycemic index such as vegetables, fresh fruits, and whole grains. They are digested more slowly and result in a more gradual release of glucose into the blood. This helps maintain stable sugar levels and avoid undesirable insulin spikes.

It can't be stressed enough, but adopting an active lifestyle is important. Regular exercise can help regulate our blood sugar by increasing insulin sensitivity. By combining a balanced diet with regular physical activity, we can maintain optimal sugar levels in our body.

Let's move beyond technical discussions and delve into the essence of what truly giving up sugar means and its transformative effects.

Imagine starting each day with clear and constant energy, without the usual roller coaster caused by blood sugar spikes and falls. This is one of the first gifts of a sugar-free life. Not only do you say goodbye to afternoon slumps, but you welcome improved focus, capable of carrying you through busy days without the exhaustion sugar leaves in its wake.

Speaking of blood sugar, did you know that by reducing your sugar intake, you give your body a chance to rebalance its natural mechanisms ? This means fewer risks of developing health issues related to high sugar levels, such as type 2 diabetes or cardiovascular disorders. It's akin to giving your body back the reins of its own health.

And that's not all. The impact goes far beyond blood sugar numbers. Your mood improves, as fluctuations in sugar levels are closely linked to our emotional states. A low-sugar diet promotes emotional stability, reducing the risks of experiencing sudden irritability or unexplained mood dips.

Physically, the benefits are just as tangible. A controlled sugar diet helps maintain a healthy weight, making the goal of weight loss less daunting and more sustainable. Your skin will thank you too; less sugar often means less inflammation, resulting in clearer and brighter skin.

But the real magic lies in the subtle changes to your everyday life. Imagine savoring a meal and truly tasting every ingredient because your taste buds aren't overwhelmed by sugar. Think of the extra energy you could invest in your passions, hobbies, or simply enjoying a more active life with loved ones. This is a regained freedom, that of no longer being a slave to sugary cravings but rather master of your food choices and, by extension, your health.

In sum, eliminating sugar from your diet isn't just a dietary decision; it's an open door to a more balanced, energetic, and serene life. It's choosing to take deep care of oneself, to respect your body, and to offer it the best fuel possible.

Chapter 9 : Sugar and longevity

The aging process is an inevitable aspect of human life. However, recent discoveries in the field of nutrition suggest that our diet could play a crucial role in how we age. Specifically, excessive sugar consumption has been linked to various detrimental effects on health, including premature aging.

Sugar, apart from its pleasing sweet taste, is known to trigger a cascade of reactions in our bodies. When we consume sugar-rich foods, our blood sugar levels rise rapidly, leading to a release of insulin, the hormone responsible for regulating our blood sugar.

However, when this regulation is constantly challenged due to a high-sugar diet, our bodies may become resistant to insulin, resulting in the development of metabolic disorders such as type 2 diabetes.

In addition to these health risks, excessive sugar consumption has also been linked to issues of premature aging. Sugar can trigger a process called glycation, during which sugar molecules bind to proteins in our bodies, forming structures called advanced glycation end products (AGEs). AGEs can damage the proteins that support the structure of our skin, thus promoting the appearance of wrinkles and fine lines.

Furthermore, consistent sugar consumption can also promote chronic inflammation, a key factor in the aging process. Chronic inflammation has been associated with a variety of age-related diseases, including heart diseases, neurodegenerative diseases such as Alzheimer's disease, and even certain types of cancer.

Beyond these well-documented effects, it is essential to highlight the psychological and behavioral impact of sugar consumption on our overall well-being, which in turn, plays a significant role in our aging process.

Sugar overconsumption not only has physical repercussions but also affects our mental and emotional health. Studies have shown that high levels of sugar in the diet can influence our mood, contributing to an increase in cases of depression and anxiety. This cycle of emotional highs and lows can make us more likely to seek comfort in food, creating a vicious cycle that is difficult to break.

Moreover, sedentary behavior, often associated with sugar-rich dietary habits, can exacerbate the situation.

Regular physical activity is a crucial pillar for keeping our bodies fit and our minds sharp as we age. Exercise not only burns calories but also stimulates the production of beneficial brain chemicals like endorphins and helps combat the detrimental effects of oxidative stress, another key factor in aging.

By adopting dietary habits that prioritize nutrient quality over sugar quantity, we not only promote healthier physical aging but also mental well-being. It involves choosing foods that nourish our bodies and support our brain function, thereby improving our overall quality of life. Foods rich in omega-3 fatty acids, antioxidants, and fiber can contribute to a robust nervous system and a healthy heart, essential for graceful aging.

Water also plays a crucial role in maintaining our health and should be a priority in our daily diet. Adequate hydration is vital for the optimal functioning of all our bodily systems. It helps eliminate toxins, maintain skin elasticity, and support cognitive health, all of which contribute to healthy aging.

Finally, establishing quality sleep is fundamental. Sugar, by disrupting our sleep cycles, can deprive us of the restorative benefits of a full night's sleep. Sleep plays a vital role in cellular regeneration and repairing the daily damage our bodies endure, in addition to consolidating our memory and regulating our mood.

In conclusion, the path to healthy and fulfilling aging is multifaceted, involving a balanced diet, regular physical activity, proper hydration, and restful sleep.

Reducing our sugar consumption is not only beneficial for slowing down the physical aging process but also a holistic strategy for improving our mental and emotional well-being. Thus, by making conscious decisions about our diet and lifestyle, we can positively influence the quality and duration of our lives.

Chapter 10 : Living a sugar-free life after the challenge

Learn how to maintain a sugar-free diet long-term and discover tips for integrating this transformation into your daily lifestyle.

Congratulations ! You've successfully completed the one-month sugar-free challenge, and you're surely feeling proud of your accomplishment. Now, you might be wondering how to sustain this sugar-free diet in the long run and incorporate these new habits into your daily life. Don't worry, we're here to guide you !

The first thing to realize is that transitioning to a sugar-free life isn't just about a one-month challenge. It's a real lifestyle change that requires determination and patience. You've managed to eliminate sugar for a month, but now it's time to find a balance for the rest of your life.

First and foremost, it's important to continue reading food labels carefully. Be vigilant and avoid processed foods as much as possible. Opt for fresh and natural foods, and prepare your own meals whenever possible. This will allow you to control the amount of sugar you consume and become aware of the composition of your diet.

It's also essential to identify traps you might fall into during this transition. Sugar can be addictive, so it's normal to experience cravings from time to time. Be prepared to deal with these cravings and find healthy alternatives to satisfy your palate. For example, you can choose fresh fruits or snacks made from nuts and seeds.

Another tip is to gradually integrate new sugar-free recipes into your daily routine.

There are many online resources that offer delicious sugar-free meal and dessert ideas. Try cooking some of them each week, and you'll quickly realize that you don't have to deprive yourself to eat healthily.

However, remember that complete sugar elimination isn't always necessary. It's entirely possible to consume sugar occasionally, as long as it remains moderate and within the framework of a balanced diet. Don't punish yourself for a small indulgence now and then, but be mindful not to fall back into old patterns of sugar overconsumption.

Finally, take advantage of this new way of eating to share your discoveries with your loved ones. Invite them to try new sugar-free recipes with you and share the benefits you've experienced from this transformation. You might be surprised at how inspiring it can be for those around you to also adopt a healthier diet.

Now that you've laid the foundation for integrating a sugar-free diet into your daily life, let's dive deeper into the long-term benefits of this transformation and explore practical tips for maintaining this new habit over the long term.

One of the major benefits of a sugar-free diet is the reduction of chronic disease risks such as type 2 diabetes, obesity, and cardiovascular diseases. By eliminating refined sugars and processed foods from your diet, you reduce your intake of empty calories and promote better blood sugar regulation. This can have a positive impact on your weight, energy levels, and overall health.

A sugar-free diet can also improve your overall health. Many people report greater mental clarity, better digestion, brighter skin, and higher energy levels after eliminating sugar from their diet. By avoiding foods high in added sugars, you allow your body to better regulate itself and function optimally.

Maintaining this new habit long-term may seem challenging, but with some practical tips, you can do it.

First, continue to educate yourself about the dangers of sugar and the benefits of mindful eating. The more you understand the advantages of this transformation, the more motivated you'll be to maintain these new habits.

Next, keep a food journal to track your consumption. Note the foods you eat and their sugar content. This will help you better understand your eating habits and identify hidden sources of sugar in your diet.

It's also important to focus on other aspects of a balanced diet. Make sure you're consuming enough protein, fiber, healthy fats, and essential vitamins and minerals. A balanced and varied diet will help you stay satisfied, maintain your energy levels, and avoid sugar cravings.

Furthermore, find healthy alternatives to sugary foods. For example, if you're craving something sweet, opt for fresh fruits or snacks made from nuts and seeds. You can also experiment with natural sweeteners like stevia or maple syrup, which can be used in moderation to add a sweet touch to your dishes.

Finally, surround yourself with support. Talk about your commitment to a sugar-free diet with your loved ones and seek out groups or online communities that share your goals.

Having people who understand and support you can be extremely beneficial when you're facing moments of temptation or doubt.

In conclusion, maintaining a sugar-free diet long-term is a real lifestyle change, but it's a change that can bring many benefits to your health and quality of life.

Continue to educate yourself, track your sugar consumption, focus on a balanced diet, and find healthy alternatives to sugary foods.

Surround yourself with support and take pleasure in sharing this new way of eating with your loved ones. You're on the path to a healthier and more fulfilling life !

PROGRESS JOURNAL

Thank you for following this brief guide to quitting sugar, I hope it has been helpful to you !
Feel free to leave a review on the Amazon platform and provide constructive feedback to help improve it to the fullest.

I invite you to track your progress on the upcoming pages of your zero sugar challenge, and I wish you success in your personal goals !

9 798322 590545